Perinatal Bereavement Services in Nassau & Suffolk Counties A Guide for Families

First Edition

About this Guide

In the early moments after losing a baby, a parent may find it difficult to articulate how that separation feels. Furthermore, how can a parent think about what to do next without feeling overwhelmed? What is the right way to feel, or grieve? What is the right thing to say or do? "What is expected of me?" is question a parent might internalize. Questions such as these abound in the hearts and minds of bereaved parents.

It is not uncommon for parents to avoid learning what to do when a baby dies, until it happens, and understandably so. I too used to avoid this topic, hoping to never deal with it, that is, until I was faced with its inevitable reality. I also found that in that heavy-hearted state, it was an immensely difficult time to research and learn what I needed to know about what to do. It simply was not the ideal time, at all, to take in new information.

This guide is the product of research and personal experiences related to early child loss. Perhaps this guide could simplify some of the process for grieving parents.

If the loss of a baby happens, it is very important for parents and families to know and feel they are supported. The purpose of this guide is to make some guidance readily accessible to parents dealing with this tremendous loss. Parents can then devote their precious quality time to themselves and their families instead of being overwhelmed with searching for answers, help, and what to do next.

With sincerest condolences,
Saidah Haziz-Ramadhan

Table of Contents

Overview of Perinatal Bereavement

(It is recommended to read this guide while sitting in a quiet, comfortable space.)

When parents hoping to start or grow their family suddenly lose a baby, time seems to stop, and the weight of the world seems to fall on their saddened hearts. Then, the tears flow as the heart aches for the little one who came, and then went. It is only natural to grieve and to feel pain. Nothing else is expected of the parents at that time. We all share in the sorrow, even when you, the parent, feel alone in the experience. After all, the missing of the baby happens because the baby existed.

(Take a break and breathe slowly, focusing on each breath as you read further.)

Perinatal bereavement is about the journey to, and through, embracing the loss. There are no "one-size-fits-all" solutions to completely erase the emptiness and pain. Instead, the focus becomes, "How do I deal with what has happened?" and when the baby means so much to the parents, "How do I preserve my baby's memories forever in my heart?"

The perinatal period extends between the 20th to 28th week of pregnancy through 28 days after birth.[1, 2] Moms, Dads, and other family members experience losses before and after this period, as well. Pregnancies unexpectedly lost before 20 weeks gestations are categorized as miscarriages[3]; hence any loss after 20 weeks can categorically be a perinatal loss. Demise before birth is called fetal death, and after birth, it is called a neonatal death.[3] Parents may also experience perinatal bereavement when a newborn is placed for adoption.

Perinatal bereavement, or bereavement in general (especially before 20 weeks), also affects the mom, and family, who was not carrying a viable pregnancy.[1, 2] This includes the experience of loss after an ectopic pregnancy[1, 3], blighted ovum/anembryonic pregnancy[1, 3], pseudocyesis[2], or hydatidiform mole.[1, 2, 3] The causes that result in the loss of a baby are many, but it is important for parents to not overwhelm themselves with thoughts of blame and guilt.[4]

(Pause for a moment. Take deeper breaths, slowly inhaling and exhaling. Then continue reading.)

Parents who experience the loss of a baby may go through the stages of loss and grief, as described by renowned psychiatrist, Dr. Elisabeth Kubler-Ross in her ground-breaking book, *On Death and* Dying.[5] These stages are 1) denial and isolation, 2) anger, 3) bargaining, such as trying to negotiate a different outcome, 4) depression, and 5) acceptance. If you, the parent, go through any or all of these phases, know that it is an expected process, and through them you may soon reach the final, acceptance phase. Keep in mind; everyone grieves in their own ways.

Beyond the initial grief is learning how to cope, and beyond coping is the road to the healing and healthy closure parents need.

(Pause for another moment. Breathe. With each slow breath, relax and think of a warm, beautiful, quiet place.)

Support and Counseling Services in Nassau and Suffolk Counties

Your healthcare provider welcomes the opportunity to be your resource for information, the care coordinator for you and your baby, and the advocate for your choices and wishes. S/he will inform you of what to expect, what procedural consents need your approval, and how much time you are afforded in the process. Likewise, feel free to simply talk to her/him; s/he is there to listen now and well into the future. In addition to the healthcare provider, there are *Support Groups and Counseling Services* to assist you. A listing of these services is available on page 11 of this guide.

(In that warm special place, think about breathing in the most pleasant of scents with each inhale.
Breathe out feelings of pain and sadness with each exhale.)

Funeral Services for Perinatal Loss

An important step in the bereavement process is planning the final services for your baby. Although it may be one of the hardest things to do as a parent, it is necessary to make the arrangements. Many funeral homes will listen to your concerns and accommodate your requests. It is common practice for most, if not all, funeral homes to offer perinatal loss services.

Jessica Koth, Public Relations Manager of the *National Funeral Directors Association*, when asked about perinatal services, stated the following:

> *Funeral homes offer a wide range of perinatal services – in fact, the same kinds of services (e.g., viewing/visitation/wake, funeral, memorial services,*

*burial, cremation, etc.) that are available for older
children and adults are also available in the case of
perinatal death. Funeral homes will work with
parents to determine what kind of service will be
most meaningful to the family.*

Ms. Koth further stated:

*In terms of cost, funeral homes have a wide range of
approaches to perinatal loss. Some will offer all
services and merchandise at no cost. Other firms
provide their services at no charge and ask families
only to pay for merchandise (e.g. casket, urn).
Compared with adult merchandise, items such as a
casket or urn for a fetus or newborn are much less
expensive. Other firms offer families a discount on all
services and merchandise.*

Take a moment to locate a funeral home near you, and give
them a call. They will walk you through every step of your
baby's final arrangements. Several funeral homes in *Nassau
and Suffolk Counties* that will provide perinatal loss services
are listed on page 15 of this guide. The funeral homes listed
are members of at least one of the following reputable
organizations: Nassau-Suffolk Funeral Directors Association,
New York State (NYS) Funeral Directors Association, Inc.,
and the National Funeral Directors Association.

The Western Perinatal Bereavement Network, Inc. has
published a *Funeral Options* resource for parents to review
in the care-after-death plan of their baby. The link is
available in the *List of Online Resources for Families* section,
page 32.

(Take a break. Continue to imagine yourself in that special place, smelling the most pleasant of scents. With your eyes closed, try to touch something beautiful; a flower or plant, or run your hands through a bubbling brook. Listen to the sounds and take in the refreshing breezes as they glide like silk across your face. Breathe slowly, and open your eyes.)

Online Resources for Families

Many organizations offer online resources for families dealing with the loss of a baby. These resources offer parents the convenience of researching and revisiting the information at any time and in privacy. For your convenience, a listing of *Online Resources* is presented in this guide on page 31.

Life after the Loss

The thought of putting the loss of a baby behind you, or moving on, can be quite overwhelming for parents. Many may find that coping with the loss of a baby means learning how to live with the memories and experiences in a positive and peaceful way, instead of attempting to ignore that the experience ever took place.

Having an understanding and acceptance of the loss's place in the lives of parents doesn't negate the reality that life does continue on after the loss. This may present another set of challenging feelings, such as sadness or guilt in the parents' dedication to the deceased baby's memory. However, the loss, and life after the loss, both deserve separate yet harmonious recognitions and purposes in the lives of bereaved parents.

Families should understand there will be challenges in continuing on with life. These challenges may surface in any area of life. This is why having emotional, psychological, and spiritual support through family, friends, and counselors, means the parents do not have to face them alone. In time, the loss does become easier to cope with. However, returning to work, school, or moving on with your daily routine, may not be easy to do.

Even pregnancy after the loss may result in a flood of concerns and emotions.[3, 6] If or when parents decide to become pregnant again, it's a good decision to schedule a preconception visit.[3, 6] At this visit, the parents can discuss their concerns and ask questions. The healthcare provider will assess the mom's psychosocial readiness for the pregnancy and refer the parents for counseling, if necessary. S/he will also assess the mom's hormonal and physical health through testing and examination. Overall, the healthcare provider will check the mom for her readiness and physical ability to have a healthy pregnancy.

Beyond the mom's physical well-being, the healthcare provider will also coordinate or maintain a psychosocial and emotional support network for her, either directly or through co-management with a psychotherapist or grief counselor. Since the worries may exist through the end of the new pregnancy, the support will help the mom, and both parents, focus on relaxation, positive thoughts, and the dispelling of unnecessary worries.[6]

Furthermore, the healthcare provider may determine that the mom experiencing a pregnancy after a loss may require additional office visits and sonograms, especially later in pregnancy. S/he can offer ultrasounds, as needed, to follow the new baby's health and growth progress.[7]

The reality is life does move on, but the parent's hearts can always treasure the baby who is no longer with them. The baby's existence can have a long-term effect on the entire family, and friends, and each person may grieve and cope differently. However, with the help and support that families need in this time, they can continue to grow in strength and size, in time. Further resources on *Beyond the Loss* are available on page 34 of this guide.

(Exhale deeply and discover the smile waiting to one day emerge from your heart. Relax peacefully knowing you can revisit this special relaxation place, anytime.)

List of Support and Counseling Services for Perinatal Bereavement in Nassau and Suffolk Counties

Nassau County

The Compassionate Friends: Syosset Chapter (Plainview/Syosset)
Chapter #: 1001
Plainview North Shore Community Hospital
888 Old Country Road
Plainview, NY 11803   718.767.0904
Email: marlenesmailbox@gmail.com
Website:
http://www.compassionatefriends.org/Find_Support/Chapters/Chapter_Locator.aspx
No cost.
Group meets 3rd Friday every month

The Compassionate Friends: Rockville Centre Chapter
Chapter #: 1626
Molloy College-Wilbur Arts Bldg. (1st floor, Hayes Theatre)
1000 Hempstead Avenue
Rockville Centre, NY 11570   516.766.4682
Email: estillwell@optonline.net
Website:
www.tcfofrvc.org
No cost.
Group meets 2nd Friday every month
- *Parents meet on 1st floor, Hayes Theater*
- *Siblings 18 & up meet in basement, Room 18*

Share Guardian Angel Perinatal Support Group
88 Hampshire Drive
Farmingdale, NY 11735   516.249.0127
Email: martyk9@optonline.net
          martha@stkilianfamily.com
Website:
http://nationalshare.org/heal/sharechapters/
No cost.
Group meets 1st Friday of every month (except July).

Center for H.O.P.E., Cohen's Children Medical Center
New Hyde Park, NY   516.470.3123
516.216.5194   Bereavement Coordinator
718.470.3124   Department of Social Work
Email: sthomas@lij.edu
Website:
http://ccmc.northshorelij.com/ccmcny-for-patients-and-families/ccmcny-bereavement-the-center-for-hope
No cost.
Contact for more information about the eight-week sessions offered several times a year

Hospice Care Network: Nassau Administrative Office – The Marks Center for Caregivers
99 Sunnyside Boulevard
Woodbury, NY 11797   800.405.6731
Website:
http://www.hospicecarenetwork.org
Accepts insurance, or no cost.
Offers individual counseling for perinatal loss

Suffolk County

The Compassionate Friends: TCF of Babylon
Chapter #: 1846
Cross of Christ Lutheran Church
576 Deer Park Avenue
Babylon, NY 11702   631.724.7250
Email: gmattera36@yahoo.com
Website:
http://www.compassionatefriends.org/Find_Support/Chapt
ers/Chapter_Locator.aspx
No cost.
Group meets 1st Friday of every month

Hospice Care Network: The Fay J. Lindner Foundation Hope & Healing Center
14 Shore Lane
Bay Shore, NY 11706   631.666.6863
Website:
http://www.hospicecarenetwork.org
Accepts insurance, or no cost.
Offers individual counseling for perinatal loss

Good Shepherd Hospice
245 Old Country Road
Melville, NY 11747   631.465.6363
Email: roger.sullivan@chsli.org
Website:
http://goodshepherdhospice.chsli.org/bereavement-
services
No cost.
Offers perinatal loss groups

Hospice Care Network: The Hospice Inn
70 Pinelawn Road
Melville, NY 11747   516.832.7100
Website:
http://www.hospicecarenetwork.org
Accepts insurance, or no cost.
Offers individual counseling for perinatal loss

The Compassionate Friends: TCF Brookhaven Chapter
Chapter #: 1739
Sylvester's Church on Robinson Street (Parish Center)
68 Ohio Avenue
Medford, NY 11763   631.738.0809
Email: walter588@aol.com
Website:
http://www.compassionatefriends.org/Find_Support/Chapt
ers/Chapter_Locator.aspx
No cost.
Group meets 2nd Friday every month

The Compassionate Friends: TCF Twin Forks/Hamptons Chapter
Chapter #: 2212
East Quogue United Methodist Church
580 Montauk Highway
East Quogue, NY 11942   631.653.9444/646.894.0317
Email: marielevine2@verizon.net
Website:
http://www.compassionatefriends.org/Find_Support/Chapt
ers/Chapter_Locator.aspx
No cost.
Group meets 3rd Friday every month

List of Funeral Services for Perinatal Loss in Nassau and Suffolk Counties

Funeral homes are alphabetically listed below by town. Those with more than one location are listed together under their first listing.

Funeral Services Organizations

Nassau-Suffolk Funeral Directors Association
http://nsfda.org/1/Home.html

NYS Funeral Directors Association, Inc.
http://www.nysfda.org/

National Funeral Directors Association
http://nfda.org/funeral-service-help-line.html

Nassau County

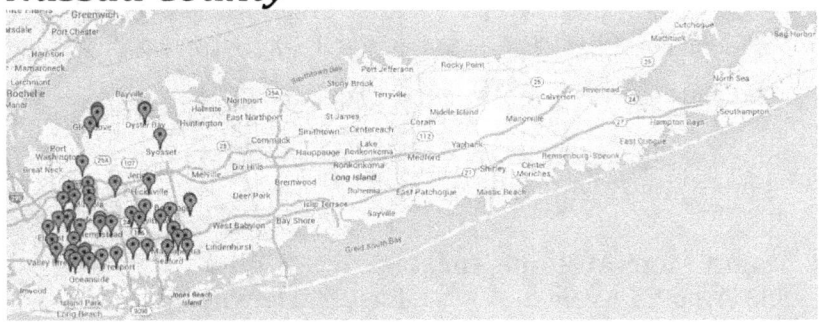

Cecere Family Funeral Home
2283 Grand Avenue   **Baldwin, NY 11510**
Phone: 516-223-4200   Fax: 516-223-9829
www.cecerefamilyfunerals.com

Fullerton Funeral Home, Inc.
769 Merrick Road   **Baldwin, NY 11510**
Phone: 516-223-1460   Fax: 516-378-7735
www.fullertonfhny.com

Clair S. Bartholomew & Son, Inc.
302 Bedford Avenue   **Bellmore, NY 11710**
Phone: 516-785-0225   Fax: 516-825-5406
www.csbartholomewandson.com

Fredrick J. Chapey & Sons Funeral Home, Inc.
20 Hicksville Rd   **Bethpage, NY 11714**
Phone: 516-731-5600   Fax: 516-731-5663
www.chapeyfamily.com

Leo F. Kearns, Inc. Funeral Homes
445 E Meadow Ave   **East Meadow, NY 11554**
Phone: 516-794-0500   Fax: 718-738-7647
www.leofkearns.com

Charles J. O'Shea Funeral Homes
2515 N. Jerusalem Ave   **East Meadow, NY 11554**
Phone: 516-826-1010   Fax: 516-826-1544
www.osheafuneral.com

603 Wantagh Avenue   **Wantagh, NY 11793**
Phone: 516-731-5550   Fax: 516-348-0164

Donza Funeral Home, Inc.
333 Atlantic Avenue   **East Rockaway, NY 11518**
Phone: 516-593-2521   Fax: 516-825-6380
www.donzafuneralhome.com

McCourt & Trudden Funeral Home
385 Main Street   **Farmingdale, NY 11735**
Phone: 516-249-1303   Fax: 516-249-0458

Arthur F. White Funeral Home, Inc.
315 Conklin Street   **Farmingdale, NY 11735**
Phone: 516-249-0336   Fax: 516-249-0369
www.arthurfwhite.com

Franklin Square Funeral Home, Inc.
42 New Hyde Park Rd   **Franklin Square, NY 11010**
Phone: 516-775-9491   Fax: 516-437-0296
www.franklinfuneralhome.net

Krauss Funeral Home, Inc.
1097 Hempstead Turnpike   **Franklin Square, NY 11010**
Phone: 516-352-2080   Fax: 516-775-1156
www.kraussfuneralhome.com

Hungerford & Clark, Inc. Funeral Home
110 Pine Street   **Freeport, NY 11520**
Phone: 516-379-3119   Fax: 516-868-6961
www.hungerfordandclark.com

Fairchild Sons Funeral Home
1201 Franklin Avenue   **Garden City, NY 11530**
Phone: 516-746-0585   Fax: 516-746-0311
www.fairchildfuneral.com

Park Funeral Chapels
2175 Jericho Turnpike   **Garden City Park, NY 11040**
Phone: 516-747-4300   Fax: 516-747-0999
www.parkfuneralchapels.com

The Whitting Funeral Home
300 Glen Cove Avenue   **Glen Head, NY 11545**
Phone: 516-671-0807   Fax: 516-676-4783
www.whitting.com

Hempstead Funeral Home: John Senko Funeral Homes
89 Peninsula Blvd.   **Hempstead, NY 11550**
Phone: 516-481-7460   Fax: 516-481-7967
www.senkofuneral.com

Jewish Memorial Chapel of Long Island – Dignity Memorial
46 Greenwich Street   **Hempstead, NY 11550**
Phone: 516-486-1060
http://www.dignitymemorialjewish.com/jewish-memorial-chapel-long-island/en-us/index.page

Vernon C. Wagner Funeral Homes: Dignity Memorial
125 Old Country Road   **Hicksville, NY 11801**
Phone: 516-935-7100   Fax: 935-0815
http://www.dignitymemorial.com/vernon-c-wagner-funeral-homes-hicksville

655 Old Country Road   **Plainview, NY 11803**
Phone: 938-4311
http://www.dignitymemorial.com/vernon-c-wagner-funeral-homes-plainview

Thomas F. Dalton Funeral Homes, Inc.
2786 Hempstead Turnpike   **Levittown, NY 11756**
Phone: 516-796-0400   Fax: 516-796-3890
www.daltonfuneralhomes.com

29 Atlantic Avenue   **Floral Park, NY 11001**
Phone: 516-354-0634   Fax: 516-354-0472

47 Jerusalem Avenue   **Hicksville, NY 11801**
Phone: 516-931-0262

125 Hillside Avenue   **New Hyde Park, NY 11040**
Phone: 516-354-0634

412 Willis Avenue   **Williston Park, NY 11596**
Phone: 354-0634

Flinch & Bruns Funeral Home, Inc.
34 Hempstead Avenue   **Lynbrook, NY 11563**
Phone: 599-3600   Fax: 599-3602
www.flinchandbruns.com

Perry Funeral Home, Inc.
118 Union Avenue   **Lynbrook, NY 11563**
Phone: 593-1111   Fax: 593-1114
www.perryfh.com

James Funeral Home: Dignity Memorial
540 Broadway   **Massapequa, NY 11758**
Phone: 516-541-4000   Fax: 516-541-4004
www.jamesfuneralhome.com

Massapequa Funeral Home, North Chapel
1050 Park Boulevard   **Massapequa Park, NY 11762**
Phone: 516-798-2500   Fax: 516-798-9380
www.massapequafuneralhome.com

Massapequa Funeral Home, South Chapel
4980 Merrick Rd   **Massapequa Park, NY 11762**
Phone: 516-798-8200   Fax: 516-798-9380
www.massapequafuneralhome.com

N. F. Walker, Inc. – Merrick Funeral Home
2039 Merrick Avenue   **Merrick, NY 11566**
Phone: 516-378-0303   Fax: 516-378-0328
www.nfwalkerfh.com

Cassidy Funeral Home, Inc.
156 Willis Avenue   **Mineola, NY 11501**
Phone: 516-746-6222   Fax: 516-746-6227
www.cassidyfh.com

New Hyde Park Funeral Home, Inc.
506 Lakeville Road   **New Hyde Park, NY 11040**
Phone: 516-352-8989   Fax: 516-352-0143
www.nhpfh.com

R. Stutzmann & Sons, Inc. – Dignity Memorial
2000 Hillside Avenue   **New Hyde Park, NY 11040**
Phone: 516-352-3434   Fax 516-352-5432
www.rstutzmannandson.com

Towers Funeral Home, Inc.
Long Beach Road   **Oceanside, NY 11572**
Phone: 516-766-0425   Fax: 516-766-9454
www.towersfuneralhomeny.com

Francis P. DeVine Funeral Home, Inc.
293 South Street   **Oyster Bay, NY 11771**
Phone: 516-922-6700   Fax: 516-922-2274
www.fpdevinefuneralhome.com

Oyster Bay Funeral Home
261 South Street   **Oyster Bay, NY 11771**
Phone: 516-922-7442   Fax: 516-922-7449
www.oysterbayfuneralhome.com

Macken Mortuary (*2 locations*)
52 Clinton Avenue   **Rockville Centre, NY 11570**
Phone: 516-766-3300   Fax: 516-766-9763
www.mackenmortuary.com

3930 Long Beach Road   **Island Park, NY 11558**
Phone: 516-431-7800

Roslyn Heights Funeral Home
75 Mineola Avenue   **Roslyn Heights, NY 11577**
Phone: 516-621-4545   Fax: 516-625-8725
www.roslynheightsfh.com

Charles G. Schmitt Funeral Home
3863 Merrick Road   **Seaford, NY 11783**
Phone: 516-785-3380   Fax: 516-826-3130
www.schmittfuneralhome.com

Hartnett Funeral Home, Inc.
561 Jerusalem Avenue   **Uniondale, NY 11553**
Phone: 516-483-9288   Fax: 516-483-9289
www.hartnettfuneralhome.com

Edward F. Lieber Funeral Homes, Inc.
266 North Central Ave   **Valley Stream, NY 11580**
Phone: 516-825-2900   Fax: 516-825-3406
www.lieberfuneralhomes.com

Barnes-Sorrentino Funeral Home, Inc.
539 Hempstead Avenue   **West Hempstead, NY 11552**
Phone: 516-481-8870   Fax: 481-8871
www.barnes-sorrentinofh.com

Donohue-Cecere Funeral Home
290 Post Avenue   **Westbury, NY 11590**
Phone: 516-333-0615   Fax: 516-333-0619
www.donohue-cecere.com

Weigand Bros. Inc.
49 Hillside Avenue   **Williston Park, NY 11596**
Phone: 516-746-4484   Fax: 516-746-6621
www.weigandbrothers.com

*PAAK Funeral Home: Specializing in Traditional Islamic Funeral Services (provides services on-site and at Masaajid and Islamic Centers in Nassau & Suffolk Counties)
58-34 Catalpa Avenue   **Ridgewood, NY 11385**
Phone: 718-418-7225   Fax: 718-418-0104
www.paakfuneral.com

Suffolk County

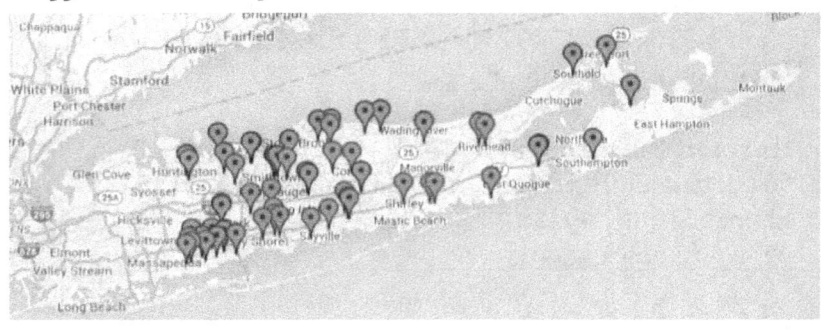

J. F. Goode Funeral Home, Inc.
545 Albany Avenue   **Amityville, NY 11701**
Phone: 631-842-6464   Fax: 631-842-6465
www.goodefuneralhome.com

Powell Funeral Home, Inc.
67 Broadway   **Amityville, NY 11701**
Phone: 631-691-0172   Fax: 631-691-2915
www.powellfh.com

Claude R. Boyd-Spencer Funeral Home – Dignity Memorial
448 W. Main Street   **Babylon, NY 11702**
Phone: 631-669-2400   Fax: 631-669-7074
www.boyd-spencer.com

Raynor & D'Andrea Funeral Homes
683 Montauk Highway   **Bayport, NY 11705**
Phone: 631-472-0122   Fax: 631-472-5410
www.raynordandrea.com   Toll free: 800-737-0017

245 Main Street   **West Sayville, NY 11796**
Phone: 631-589-2345   Fax: 631-589-5436

Masjid Darul Quran Burial Services
1514 East 3rd Avenue   **Bay Shore, NY 11706**
Phone: 631-665-9642 or 631-220-9373
www.masjiddarulquran.com/web/burialservices

*PAAK Funeral Home: Specializing in Traditional Islamic Funeral Services (provides services on-site and at Masaajid and Islamic Centers in Nassau & Suffolk Counties)
58-34 Catalpa Avenue   **Ridgewood, NY 11385**
Phone: 718-418-7225   Fax: 718-418-0104
www.paakfuneral.com

Michael J. Grant Funeral Homes, Inc.
571 Suffolk Avenue   **Brentwood, NY 11717**
Phone: 631-273-4443   Fax: 631-273-2286
www.grantfh.com

3640 Route 112   **Coram, NY 11727**
Phone: 631-696-0909   Fax: 631-273-2286

Sinnickson's Moriches Funeral Home
203 Main Street   **Center Moriches, NY 11934**
Mailing: P.O. Box 603
Phone: 631-878-0065   Fax: 631-874-3965
www.sinnicksons.com

Wesche Funeral Home, Inc.
495 Main Street   **Center Moriches, NY 11934**
Phone: 631-878-0007   Fax: 631-874-7286
www.weschefh.com

O.B. Davis Funeral Homes – Dignity Memorial
2326 Middle Country Road   **Centereach, NY 11720**
Phone: 631-585-8888   Fax: 631-585-6045
www.obdavis.com

1001 Route 25a   **Miller Place, NY 11764**
Phone: 631-744-1001   Fax: 631-744-9164

4839 Nesconset Highway   **Port Jefferson Station, NY 11776**

Phone: 631-473-0360   Fax: 631-473-8589

Thomas P. Walsh Funeral Home
60 Carleton Ave   **Central Islip, NY 11722**
Phone: 631-274-6008
www.thomaspwalshfuneralhome.com

Commack Abbey, Inc.
96 Commack Road   **Commack, NY 11725**
Phone: 631-499-4422   Fax: 631-499-5273
www.commackabbeyinc.com

D'Andrea Brothers Funeral Home – Dignity Memorial
99 Oak Street   **Copiague, NY 11726**
Phone: 631-691-5700   Fax: 631-691-6263
www.dandreabrosfuneral.com

Claude R. Boyd-Caratozzolo Funeral Home – Dignity Memorial
1785 Deer Park Avenue   **Deer Park, NY 11729**
Phone: 631-667-8614   Fax: 631-586-0205
www.boyd-caratozzolofuneralhome.com

Albrecht Bruno & O'Shea Funeral Homes
62 Carleton Avenue   **East Islip, NY 11730**
Phone: 631-581-2828   Fax: 631-581-0809
www.osheafuneral.com

Brueggemann Funeral Home of East Northport, Inc.
522 Larkfield Road   **East Northport, NY 11731**
Phone: 631-368-1235   Fax: 631-368-4372
www.brueggemannfh.com

Fredrick J. Chapey & Sons Funeral Home, Inc.
200 East Main Street   **East Islip, NY 11730**
Phone: 631-581-5600   Fax: 631-581-5151
www.chapeyfamily.com

1225 Montauk Highway   **West Islip, NY 11795**
Phone: 631-661-5644   Fax: 631-661-5672

Horton-Mathie Funeral Home
735 First Street   **Greenport, NY 11944**
Phone: 631-477-0054
www.horton-mathie.com

R. J. O'Shea, Funeral Home
94 East Montauk Highway   **Hampton Bays, NY 11946**
Phone: 631-728-3131   Fax: 631-728-3131
www.rjosheafuneralhome.com

J. Ronald Scott Funeral Home
20 Ponquoque Avenue   **Hampton Bays, NY 11946**
Phone: 631-728-3660   Fax: 631-728-3717

M. A. Connell Funeral Home
934 New York Avenue   **Huntington Station, NY**
                                           11746
Phone: 631-427-1123   Fax: 631-385-2306
www.maconnellfuneralhome.com

Overton Funeral Home, Inc.
172 Main Street   **Islip, NY 11751**
Mailing: P.O. Box 487
Phone: 631-581-5085   Fax: 631-581-2681
        631-446-2186
www.overtonfuneralhome.com

Sandles Funeral Home
98 Carleton Avenue   **Islip Terrace, NY 11752**
Phone: 631-581-9242   Fax: 631-581-3284

Butler-Hughes Funeral Home
69 Indian Head Road   **Kings Park, NY 11754**
Phone: 631-269-4555   Fax: 631-269-6344
Toll Free: 888-892-1771
www.butler-hughesfuneralhome.com

Clayton Funeral Home
25 Meadow Road   **Kings Park, NY 11754**
Phone: 631-269-6421   Fax: 631-269-6410
www.claytonkingspark.com

Moloney's Lake Funeral Home & Cremation Center
132 Ronkonkoma Avenue   **Lake Ronkonkoma, NY**
                                                 11779

Phone: 631-588-1515   Fax: 631-588-9126
www.moloneyfh.com

Moloney's Port Jefferson Station Funeral Home
523 Route 112   **Port Jefferson Station, NY**
                                                 11776

Phone: 631-473-3800

Moloney's Bohemia Funeral Home
120 Lakeland Avenue   **Bohemia, NY 11716**
Phone: 631-589-1500

Moloney's Hauppauge Funeral Home
840 Wheeler Road (Rte. 111) **Hauppauge, NY 11788**
Phone: 631-361-7500

Moloney's Holbrook Funeral Home
825 Main Street **Holbrook, NY 11741**
Phone: 631-981-7500

Moloney Funeral Home
135 Carleton Avenue **Central Islip, NY 11722**
Phone: 631-234-6000

Joseph A. Weber Funeral Home, Inc.
231 Hawkins Ave **Lake Ronkonkoma, NY 11779**

Phone: 588-9599 Fax: 588-6630
www.jaweberfuneralhome.com

Johnstons' Wellwood Funeral Home
305 N. Wellwood Avenue **Lindenhurst, NY 11757**
Phone: 631-226-2220 Fax: 631-226-2642
www.wellwoodfuneralhome.com

Lindenhurst Funeral Home
424 S. Wellwood Avenue **Lindenhurst, NY 11757**
Phone: 631-957-0300 Fax: 631-957-0306
www.lindenhurstfuneralhome.com

McManus-Lorey Funeral Home
2084 Horseblock Road **Medford, NY 11763**
Phone: 631-732-1112 Fax: 631-736-6695
www.mcmanuslorey.com

New York Atlantic Funeral Services Corp.
2084 Horse Block Rd   **Medford, NY 11763**
Phone: 631-732-0570 or   Fax: 631-732-0572
Toll free: 800-645-3722
www.nyatlanticfuneralservices.com

Nolan & Taylor-Howe Funeral Home
5 Laurel Avenue   **Northport, NY 11768**
Phone: 754-2400   Fax: 261-6190
Toll Free: 800-261-8338
www.nolantaylorhowefh.com

Robertaccio Funeral Home, Inc.
85 Medford Avenue   **Patchogue, NY 11772**
Phone: 631-475-7000   Fax: 631-475-5831
www.robertacciofuneralhome.com

Ruland Funeral Home
500 North Ocean Avenue   **Patchogue, NY 11772**
Phone: 631-475-0098   Fax: 631-475-1270
www.therulandfuneralhome.com

Casimir Funeral Home – Dignity Memorial
4839 Nesconset Highway   **Port Jefferson Station, NY 11776**
Phone: 631-473-0360   Fax: 631-473-8589
www.casimirfuneralhome.com

Reginald H. Tuthill Funeral Home
406 East Main Street   **Riverhead, NY 11901**
Phone: 631-727-2403   Fax: 631-727-2404
www.rhtuthillfuneralhome.com

Rocky Point Funeral Home
603 Rte. 25A   **Rocky Point, NY 11778**
Phone: 631-744-9000   Fax: 631-821-9050
www.rockypointfuneralhome.com

Joseph A. Weber Funeral Home
231 Hawkins Avenue   **Ronkonkoma, NY 11779**
Phone: 631-588-9599   Fax: 631-588-6630
www.jaweberfuneralhome.com

Yardley & Pino Funeral Home, Inc.
91 Hampton Street   **Sag Harbor, NY 11963**
Phone: 631-725-0251   Fax: 631-725-0256
www.yardleypino.com

Giove Funeral Home
1000 Middle Country Road   **Selden, NY 11784**
Phone: 631-732-1800   Fax: 631-698-0266
www.giovefuneralhome.com

Bryant Funeral Home, Inc.
411 Old Town Rd   **Setauket, NY 11733**
Mailing: P.O. Box 705
Phone: 631-473-0082   Fax: 631-473-0927
www.bryantfh.com

The Shelter Island Funeral Home
23 West Neck Road   **Shelter Island, NY 11964**
Mailing: P.O. Box 944
Phone: 631-749-2212   Fax: 631-765-4056
www.defriestgrattan.com

Roma Funeral Home
539 William Floyd Parkway   **Shirley, NY 11967**
Phone: 631-281-0800   Fax: 631-281-6435
www.romafuneralhome.com

De Friest-Grattan Funeral Homes
51400 Route 25   **Southold, NY 11971**
Mailing: PO Box 508
Phone: 631-765-3850   Fax: 631-765-4056
www.defriestgrattan.com

St. James Funeral Home, Inc.
829 Middle Country Road   **St. James, NY 11780**
Phone: 631-584-7200
www.stjamesfuneralhome.com

Brockett Funeral Home, Inc.
203 Hampton Road   **Southampton, NY 11968**
Phone: 631-283-0822   Fax: 631-283-0883
www.brockettfuneralhome.com

Alexander-Tuthill Funeral Home
6447 Route 25A   **Wading River, NY 11792**
Mailing: P.O. Box 695
Phone: 631-929-4111   Fax: 631-929-0434
Toll-Free: 877-929-4111
www.alexandertuthillfuneralhome.com

Noce Funeral Home, Inc.
189 Route 109   **West Babylon, NY 11704**
Phone: 631-422-0100   Fax: 631-422-0101
www.nocefuneralhome.com

Follett & Werner Funeral Home
60 Mill Road   **Westhampton Beach, NY**
                                      11978

Phone: 631-288-1231   Fax: 631-288-6945
www.follettandwerner.com

Claude R. Boyd-Spencer Funeral Homes – Dignity Memorial
255 Higbie Lane   **West Islip, NY 11795**
Phone: 631-669-8338   Fax: 631-482-8088
http://www.dignitymemorial.com/claude-r-boyd-spencer-funeral-homes-west-islip

List of Online Resources for Families

Perinatal Bereavement Resources

The following links from organizations, including the March of Dimes, Western New York Perinatal Bereavement Network, and The Compassionate Friends, offer practical advice and information for parents and their families during their loss and grieving process.

Types of Losses

When Pregnancy Loss Happens:
http://www.marchofdimes.org/loss/pregnancy-loss.aspx

The Loss of a Baby:
www.marchofdimes.org/loss/the-loss-of-a-baby.aspx

Early Losses:
http://www.wnypbn.org/images/Early_Losses_-_Miscarriage.pdf

Stillbirth:
http://www.wnypbn.org/images/Stillbirth.pdf

Stillbirth:
http://www.marchofdimes.org/loss/stillbirth.aspx

Neonatal Death:
http://www.marchofdimes.org/loss/neonatal-death.aspx

Early Infant Death:
http://www.wnypbn.org/images/Early_Infant_Death.pdf

Losing an Only Child:
http://www.wnypbn.org/images/Losing_an_Only_Child.pdf

Death of Multiples:
http://www.wnypbn.org/images/Death_of_Multiples.pdf

Newborn Loss: Frequently Asked Questions:
http://www.marchofdimes.org/loss/newborn-loss.aspx#QATabAlt

Pregnancy & Infant Loss and Infertility Support – Long Island. Information and Counseling on Reproductive Issues and Grief:
http://longislandpregnancyandinfantloss.com/pregnancy-and-infant-loss/

Funeral Options

Funeral Options:
http://www.wnypbn.org/images/Funeral_Options.pdf

Grieving

You Are Not Alone:
http://www.compassionatefriends.org/Find_Support/Personal-Note/To_the_Newly_Bereaved.aspx

Self-Help:
http://www.wnypbn.org/images/Self-Help%20(1).pdf

Dealing with Your Grief:
www.marchofdimes.org/loss/dealing-with-your-grief.aspx

The Grieving Process:
http://www.wnypbn.org/images/The_Grieving_Process.pdf

Dealing with the Unexpected:
http://www.marchofdimes.org/loss/dealing-with-the-unexpected.aspx

Coping with the Death of Your Baby:
www.marchofdimes.org/loss/dealing-with-grief.aspx

Helping Yourself Heal When a Baby Dies:
http://griefwords.com/index.cgi?action=page&page=articles%2Fhelping5.html&site_id=37

Men & Women Grieve Differently:
http://www.wnypbn.org/images/Men_&_Women_Grieve_Differently.pdf

Father's Grief:
http://www.wnypbn.org/images/Father%27s_Grief%20(1).pdf

Single Parent Grief:
http://www.wnypbn.org/images/Single_Parent_Grief%20(1).pdf

Dealing with Others as You Grieve:
www.marchofdimes.org/loss/dealing-with-others-as-you-grieve.aspx

Children-Sibling Grief:
http://www.wnypbn.org/images/Children-Sibling_Grief.pdf

Grandparents:
http://www.wnypbn.org/images/Grandparents.pdf

Friends & Family:
http://www.wnypbn.org/images/Friends_&_FAmily.pdf

Fredrick J. Chapey & Sons: Griefwords Library by Dr. Alan
Wolfelt, Ph.D.:
http://www.griefwords.com/library/active/chapeyfamily.as
p

Inner Health Studio – Easy Relaxation Techniques:
http://www.innerhealthstudio.com/

Beyond the Loss

Remembering Your Baby:
http://www.marchofdimes.org/loss/remembering-your-baby.aspx

From Hurt to Healing:
http://www.marchofdimes.org/loss/from-hurt-to-healing.aspx

Returning to Work:
http://www.wnypbn.org/images/Returning_to_Work.pdf

Subsequent Pregnancy:
http://www.wnypbn.org/images/Subsequent_Pregnancy.pd
f

Resources and Readings

Care Card:
http://www.wnypbn.org/images/New%20Care%20Card.pdf

When a Child Dies – A Guide for Family and Friends:
http://www.caringinfo.org/files/public/brochures/When_A_Child_Dies.pdf

Helpful Articles and References:
http://www.wnypbn.org/images/Helpful_Articles_&_References.pdf

Useful Forms

Fetal Death Record:
http://www.wnypbn.org/images/DOH-3667.pdf

Certificate of Stillbirth:
http://www.wnypbn.org/images/CSB_doh-5056.pdf

Additional Online Resources

Angel Babies Forever Loved and Missed:
https://www.facebook.com/AngelBabiesForever

First Candle - Grief Support Hotline: 800-221-7437
http://www.sidsalliance.org/

First Candle – Online Support Group:
www.firstcandle.org

GriefNet Neonatal Loss Support Email Group:
(Choose "neonatal-loss" in the Support Group section of the form)
http://griefnet.org/support/SGform.html

Twinless Twins Support Group:
http://www.twinlesstwins.org/

March of Dimes:
www.marchofdimes.com

Bereaved Parents of the USA:
http://www.bereavedparentsusa.org/

The Compassionate Friends – Supporting Family After a Child Dies:
http://www.compassionatefriends.org/Find_Support.aspx

Share: Pregnancy & Infant Loss Support – Find Share Chapters Across the Country:
http://nationalshare.org/heal-2/sharechapters/

Together for Short Lives – Help for Families:
http://www.togetherforshortlives.org.uk/families/faqs

Perinatal Hospice and Palliative Care – A Gift of Time:
http://perinatalhospice.org/Home_Page.html

The Compassionate Friends, Inc.:
www.compassiontefriends.org

Mothers in Sympathy and Support (M.I.S.S.):
www.missfoundation.org

A Source of Help in Airing and Resolving Experiences (SHARE):
www.selfhelp.prairienet.org

Aiding a Mother and Father Experiencing Neonatal Death (AMEND):
www.amendgroup.com

Grief Recovery: The Action Program for Moving Beyond Loss:
www.grief-recovery.com

References

1. Cunningham F, Leveno KJ, Bloom SL, Spong CY, Dashe JS, Hoffman BL, Casey BM, Sheffield JS. eds. Williams Obstetrics, Twenty-Fourth Edition. New York, NY: McGraw-Hill; 2013.

2. Taber's® Cyclopedic Medical Dictionary. 22nd ed. Donald Venes MDMSJFACP, editor. Philadelphia, PA: F. A. Davis Company; 2013.

3. King TL, Brucker MC, Kriebs JM, Fahey JO, Gegor CL, Varney H. Varney's midwifery, Fifth Edition. Burlington: Jones & Bartlett; 2015.

4. Thorstensen KA. Midwifery Management of First Trimester Bleeding and Early Pregnancy Loss. The J Midwifery Wom Heal. 2000;45(6):481-497.

5. Kubler-Ross E. On death and dying. (First Scribner Classics Edition 1997). New York, NY: Scribner; 1969. http://books.google.com/books?id=zb-ZNYFUXhsC&pg=PA25&source=gbs_toc_r&cad=3#v=onepage&q&f=false. Accessed April 7, 2015.

6. Lee L, McKenzie-McHarg K, Horsch A. Women's Decision Making and Experience of Subsequent Pregnancy Following Stillbirth. J Midwifery Wom Heal. 2013;58(4):431-439.

7. Rowland A, Goodnight WH. Fetal Loss: Addressing the Evaluation and Supporting the Emotional Needs of Parents. The J Midwifery Wom Heal. 2009;54(3):241-248.